Michelle Bianchi de Moraes
Fernando Vagner Raldi

Assessment of vertebral bone age in individuals with Down Syndrome

Michelle Bianchi de Moraes
Fernando Vagner Raldi

Assessment of vertebral bone age in individuals with Down Syndrome

Imprint

Any brand names and product names mentioned in this book are subject to trademark, brand or patent protection and are trademarks or registered trademarks of their respective holders. The use of brand names, product names, common names, trade names, product descriptions etc. even without a particular marking in this work is in no way to be construed to mean that such names may be regarded as unrestricted in respect of trademark and brand protection legislation and could thus be used by anyone.

Cover image: www.ingimage.com

This book is a translation from the original published under ISBN 978-613-9-61483-7.

Publisher:
Sciencia Scripts
is a trademark of
Dodo Books Indian Ocean Ltd. and OmniScriptum S.R.L publishing group

120 High Road, East Finchley, London, N2 9ED, United Kingdom
Str. Armeneasca 28/1, office 1, Chisinau MD-2012, Republic of Moldova, Europe
Printed at: see last page
ISBN: 978-620-7-63117-9

Table of contents:

Vertebral bone age assessment in individuals with Down Syndrome

Chapter 1

1 INTRODUCTION

Down's syndrome is characterized by intellectual impairment and numerous physical anomalies resulting from trisomy 21. Langdon Down, in 1866, made the first description of individuals with the characteristics of trisomy 21, under the name Mongolian idiocy, which fell into disuse due to the recommendation of the World Health Organization (WHO), and was later called Down syndrome[6].

Individuals with this syndrome are characterized by mild to moderate intellectual impairment, as well as other clinical alterations such as: muscular hypotonia, oblique palpebral fissure, large hands and short fingers, cardiac deficiencies, microcephaly, short stature, dysplastic ears with low implantation, patella-femoral instability, atlanto-axial instability, joint hyper-extension, increased retinal vascularization, immune deficiency, cleft tongue, dental anomalies, open bite, high incidence of periodontal disease and low prevalence of caries[26].

Human growth and development are gradual processes and are associated with various physical changes. Chronological age, i.e. the period of time between fertilization and the individual's current age, is not a sufficient criterion for analyzing growth and development and needs to be related to other biological indices.

The assessment of human development in dentistry is mainly based on bone maturation and tooth mineralization. A large part of professional activity is focused on interpreting factors related to the growth and facial development of individuals. This information justifies the constant use of panoramic, hand and wrist radiographs to analyze dental and bone development respectively. They are used with greater intensity in some specialties of dentistry since they are directly related to human growth[2].

Guzzi and Carvalho[14] pointed out that assessing skeletal maturity using hand and wrist radiographs is one of the complementary tests used for diagnosis and orthodontic treatment planning.

Concern about protecting patients from the use of ionizing radiation is increasingly widespread in the dental profession. This can be seen in the incessant search for new methods of assessing human development. To the detriment of this, there is currently the possibility of using the cervical vertebrae to check bone development, since teleradiography, being an examination of choice in the orthodontic and facial orthopedics protocol and its visualization being possible in this examination, could replace hand and wrist radiography. This would imply a reduction in the ionizing radiation received by the individual undergoing radiographic examinations, which would ensure control of the biological effects[7] .

Currently, the method devised by Lamparski[20] and modified by Hassel and Farman[17] , which analyzes bone maturation from the second to the fourth cervical vertebra, is a very practical and reliable alternative for use as a bone age estimator. According to O'Reilly and Yanniello[29] , the study of bone development and age through the cervical vertebrae is valid and reproducible when compared to the method that uses hand and wrist radiographs.

Bearing in mind that the bone development of children with Down's syndrome varies when compared to those without the syndrome, new studies on Down's syndrome patients should be carried out in order to provide further clarification and improve the quality of life of these individuals.

Chapter 2

2 LITERATURE REVIEW

To make things easier to understand, the subjects have been covered separately in topics.

2.1 Down Syndrome

Coelho et al.[6], in 1982, showed that the first description of the characteristics of children with trisomy 21 occurred in 1866, and at the time it was called Mongolian idiocy, due to the physical similarities of the affected individuals to those of the Mongolian race. It later became known as Down's syndrome, which is also known as trisomy 21. It is of great interest to dental surgeons because it is associated with various craniofacial and dental anomalies. It is characterized by mild to moderate intellectual impairment and numerous physical anomalies, resulting from the existence of extra genetic material on chromosome 21.

Rey et al.[31] in 1991 concluded that Down syndrome patients have almond-shaped orbital forms, and their craniofacial development differs in terms of maxillary growth rates and pneumatization of the maxillary sinuses. With regard to the occlusion of the arches, important occlusal disharmonies are observed, such as Angle class III occlusion and also anterior and/or posterior crossbite, as well as anterior open bite and with regard to dental aspects, congenital absences, anodontia, microdontia, delayed root formation, hypoplasia and fusion, as well as delayed tooth eruption, are observed in both dentitions.

Ferreira et al.[9] , in 1993, using 80 panoramic radiographs of male and female Down syndrome patients, concluded that they had statistically non-significant dental agenesis:

a) between the upper teeth of males compared to females;

b) between the lower teeth of males compared to females.

There were statistically significant dental agenesis when comparing the upper and lower arches in males and females. The greatest number of agenetic teeth, in descending order, are the upper lateral incisors, upper second premolars, lower lateral incisors and lower second premolars. Male carriers of the syndrome show agenesis of practically only the upper lateral incisors.

Ferreira et al.[10] , in 1998, clinically and radiographically examined 1,988 teeth from 71 male and female leucoderma patients with Down syndrome, 38 females and 33 males, aged between 9 and 36 years. They observed that:

1) there was no gyroversion in the central incisors and molars, both upper and lower, in males and females;

2) the premolars of male and female subjects, both upper and lower, were the teeth that showed the most gyroversions, followed by the canines;

3) the highest percentage of teeth with gyroversion was found in females.

Sannomiya et al.[33] , in 1998, obtained a sample of 81 children with Down's syndrome, aged between 6 and 15 years, who underwent radiographic incidences of the hand and wrist on the left side. The method used to assess bone age was to compare the radiographs of the hand and wrist with the standards set out in the Greulich and Pyle atlas[15] (1959). From the results obtained, they concluded that:

1) the 120 to 155-month-old female group and the 156 to 180-month-old male group showed statistically significant differences when analyzing chronological age and bone age;

2) the Greulich and Pyle atlas[15] can be used to estimate bone age in individuals with Down syndrome, with the exception of the groups mentioned above for the respective sexes.

Aguiar[2] in 1998, in his thesis, morphometrically analyzed the carpal and metacarpal bones of children with Down's syndrome and compared them with images of the same bones of children without the syndrome, of the same age, male and female. The statistical results show that the girls with the syndrome had less bone development than the girls without the syndrome; the girls with the syndrome had less bone development than the boys who also had Down's syndrome, and the boys with the syndrome had bone development similar to the boys without the syndrome in terms of peak growth at fourteen and fifteen years of age.

Silva et al.[36] , in 2003, showed that children with Down syndrome have delayed eruption of teeth, both deciduous and permanent, compared to phenotypically normal children. The deciduous dentition of children with Down syndrome is completed between 3 and 4 years of age, and the upper and lower permanent lateral incisors show delayed eruption.

Papich et al.[30], in 2005, studied chewing and dental occlusion in people with Down's syndrome, observing that they have inadequate chewing, characterized by a lateral bite of the food, lack of lip velamentum, vertical mandibular mobility and altered tongue mobility. All of these aspects, together with the altered occlusion and bite found in these individuals, mean that there is a need for adapted feeding.

Sannomiya et al.[34], in 2005, verified the existence of a correlation between chronological and estimated bone ages in patients with Down's syndrome, between 5 and 16 years of age, using radiographs of the left hand and wrist evaluated using the Eklof and Ringertz method, using the Radiocef program from Radiomemory (Belo Horizonte, Brazil). The results showed that the chronological age is two years and five months higher than the estimated bone age and, therefore, the index proposed by Eklof and Ringertz is not reliable for assessing these parameters in individuals with Down syndrome.

Hala et al. in 2016 showed closer values and less discordance between dental age (DA) and chronological age (CA) than skeletal age (SA) and chronological age (CA) for individuals with and without Down syndrome (DS). Based on this evidence, it seems fair to suggest that DA, using Nolla's method, is more accurate than SA, using Greulich and Pyle's method. More caution is needed when estimating age for individuals with DS, since they show much more variation than individuals without DS. However, none of the methods is absolutely accurate in estimating AC for individuals with DS. It is believed that the combination of the SA and DA variables could represent a significant improvement in the prediction of AC for individuals with DS, reducing the possibility of errors.

2.2. Hand and wrist bone development

Greulich and Pyle[15], in 1959, presented patterns of bone development in the hand and wrist of 133 American children aged between 0 and 18 years. The aim of the study was to demonstrate that children without the syndrome show variations in the speed of maturation according to age. The authors found marked age differences for the onset of ossification centers. This observation suggests that, at the time of the onset of ossification, a center may be subject to influences that temporarily affect its growth rate, but which may not affect the overall bone development process.

Tanner and Whitehouse[37] in 1959 developed a method in which each ossification center selected would receive a corresponding score, the sum of the scores would determine a value which, taken from the table created by the author, would indicate bone age. This method was based on a sample of 1500 English children.

Acheson et al.[1] , in 1966, estimated the intrinsic error of the Greulich and Pyle[15] and Tanner and Whitehouse[37] (TW1) methods, using 50 hand and wrist radiographs of 25 boys and 25 girls, aged between 2 and 18 years. The radiographs were assessed twice by 6 observers, who were instructed to study the introduction to the atlas by Greulich and Pyle[15] and the text accompanying the TW1 method. After analyzing the results, it was found that the bone ages estimated by the Greulich and Pyle Atlas[15] were lower than those determined by the TW1 method by approximately one year. The authors concluded that the TW1 method generates less variation than the Greulich and Pyle Atlas[15] , providing smaller systematic errors. According to the authors, the differences between the two methods in estimating bone age can be attributed to the fact that the populations used to design these systems developed under different environmental circumstances, which led to maturity at different times.

In 1967 Eklöf and Ringertz[8] proposed a method based on linear measurements of the following areas of the hand and wrist: width of the distal epiphysis of the radius, length of the capitate, width of the capitate, length of the hamate, width of the hamate, length of the 2nd, 3rd and 4th metacarpal bones and length of the proximal phalanges of the 2nd and 3rd fingers. Each ossification center is measured and this value is compared to a table according to gender. The values found in the table are added up, their average subtracted and the bone age obtained. This method was based on Swedish children aged between 1 and 15 years.

Kimura[18] in 1975 related chronological and bone ages, discussing the growth of the second metacarpal bone, based on hand and wrist X-rays, in 499 Japanese boys and 424 girls, aged between 1 and 18 years. He found that the width of the bone progresses in parallel in both sexes, until adolescence, when there is a more rapid increase in boys. The length and width indices are always higher in boys, but the differences between the sexes become significant after adolescence. As a result, two differences between the sexes are identified for growth and development of the second metacarpal in pre- and post-adolescence. In pre-adolescence, girls appear to be more advanced in their development, while in post-adolescence, there is a greater increase in length in boys, which seems to be the characteristic of the differences between the sexes.

Tavano[40] in 1976 compared the estimation of bone age determined by the indices of Greulich and Pyle (1959); Tanner and Whitehouse (1959); Schmid and Moll (1960) and Eklof and Ringertz (1967) in 590 Brazilian male and female leucodermic children aged between 3 and 17 years. The Tanner and Whitehouse (1959) and Schmid and Moll (1960) indices were used in two ways, complete and simplified, and compared with each other. Through an analysis of the applicability of these indices in relation to the population studied, the author made considerations for each index. In the American Greulich and Pyle index, they observed precociousness in Brazilian children at the youngest ages, with the opposite occurring for adolescents; for the English Tanner and Whitehouse index, in males, there was precociousness in bone development at the youngest ages and delay at the oldest, and the opposite for females. The German Schmid and Moll index showed early bone development in males and the opposite in females. For the Swedish index, Eklof and Ringertz found delayed bone development in males and females at younger ages, and the opposite for adolescents. The author concluded that there was statistical significance for all the correlations studied, demonstrating the existence of a strong relationship between the indices and chronological age. Among the indices studied, the Eklof and Ringertz index showed the highest correlation with chronological age (0.98 for males and 0.97 for females).

Marshall[21] stated in 1976 that the female sex is, on average, two and a half years ahead of boys, although it varies widely in intensity and duration from one youngster to another. The pubertal growth spurt generally lasts the same length of time for males and females. The years of adolescence transform a child into an adult, capable of performing all the biological functions of maturity. The amount of bone mass decreases, with the fusion of the epiphyses and diaphyses and the falling out of the deciduous teeth.

In 1983 Tanner et al.[38] , presented a revised version of their method described in 1959, called Tanner and Whitehouse (TW2). In this system, there were separate maturity indices for the carpal bones, and for the radius, ulna and short bones (RUS), while retaining the twenty-bone method (TW2-20). In this version, the final stages of maturity of the radius and ulna, as well as some carpal bones, were excluded because the authors considered the assessment to be difficult and unreliable. The skeletal maturity score tables were separated by gender and the mathematical procedure for assigning maturity stage values was refined. A study was carried out in 1990 by Freitas et al.[12] , who observed that in males and females there was statistical significance in the correlations between chronological age, pubertal age, stature, bone and dental age.

According to Moyers[28] in 1991, growth is defined as changes in the quantity of living substance. The quantitative aspect of biological development is measured in units of time (weight, height). Development can be defined as the series of events in normal sequence between fertilization of the egg and the adult state. Maturation means full development, the stabilization of the adult state effected by growth and development.

Moraes et al.[23] , in 1994, carried out a study to compare bone age indices with chronological age in a sample of 222 male and female leucoderma individuals from the city of Sao José dos Campos, aged between 3.5 and 14 years, divided into groups of five with a chronological age interval of 6 months. Carpal radiographs were taken and analyzed using the Greulich and Pyle method[15] to obtain bone age, which was then compared with chronological age. The results showed a delay in bone age for both males and females, although females were earlier than males. The authors concluded that the foreign developmental standards used to estimate bone age are not adapted to Brazilian children, leading to inaccurate results.

Moraes[24] , in 1995, carried out a study using X-rays of the face, where he found that there was an asymmetry in the development of the right and left hands when calculating bone age. This asymmetry was not significant, allowing either hand to be used without any difference in bone age.

In 1997, Moraes[25] , using a sample of 244 males and females aged between 84 and 191 months and panoramic and hand and wrist radiographs of the same individual, observed that there was a positive correlation between the mean chronological, dental and bone ages, when grouped according to the stages of the pubertal growth spurt.

In 2000, Guzzi and Carvalho[14] estimated the bone maturity in hand and wrist radiographs of 95 Brazilian male and female children between 9 years and 1 month and 16 years and 8 months of chronological age. The Greulich and Pyle atlas[15] (1959) was used to estimate bone age, and growth curves were also constructed to determine the age of the pubertal growth spurt. The authors observed that the estimated bone age was higher than the chronological age in females and lower in males. The average age at which the pubertal growth spurt occurs was 11 years and 9 months for girls and 13 years and 11 months for boys.

Haiter Neto et al. in 2000 checked the accuracy of the Greulich and Pyle[15] (1959) and Tanner and Whitehouse[37] (1959) methods for determining bone age. The sample consisted of 160 female and male individuals with chronological ages ranging from six years and ten months to 14 years and nine months. They were divided into groups of ten individuals - half for each sex - and for periods of six months between them. They found that there was an overestimation of age for the females and an underestimation for the males. They also found that the linear correlation between the two ages was positive and significant at 1%, making it almost perfect. Even though they obtained a high correlation, they pointed out that it is necessary to calculate the straight line equation in order to adjust the methods used to the Brazilian population. They concluded that the methods showed a high correlation with chronological age, but that it is necessary to make a correction in order to apply them to other populations.

In 2003 Tanner et al.[39] modified the Tanner and Whitehouse method[38] (TW2), calling it Tanner and Whitehouse[39] (TW3). The system of twenty bones was abolished, leaving only RUS and CARPAIS.

The stages and scores assigned to the hand and wrist bones remained unchanged, but the bone ages were modified. The adult height prediction equations were also modified.

Kurita[19] in 2004 analyzed dental and bone age in individuals from Ceará. To estimate bone age, the Greulich and Pyle[15] (1959), Eklöf and Ringertz[8] (1967) and Tanner and Whitehouse[38] (2003) methods were used on a sample of 360 individuals aged between 82 and 189 months, divided into 18 age groups according to chronological age. To estimate bone age using the Greulich and Pyle method, the radiographs of each patient's hand and wrist were compared with the standardized radiographic plates from the Greulich and Pyle Atlas. As for the TW3 (RUS) method, scores are obtained according to the stage of mineralization of the ossification centers studied, and once these stages have been added up, the result obtained is transformed into bone age using the tables proposed by the authors. For Eklöf and Ringertz, a computerized method was used, using a program called Radiocef 2000, where 8 ossification centers were analyzed, obtaining 10 linear values of length and/or width. With this study, the author observed that: a) the correlation between dental and chronological ages for males showed no statistically significant differences between the methods studied; but they did show differences between the methods and chronological age; and for females there were statistical differences between the methods and between them and chronological age; b) the correlation between bone age and chronological age showed no statistically significant differences for males; and for females, the Eklöf and Ringertz method showed statistically significant differences with chronological age and the other methods.

Damian et al.[7] , in 2006, used 210 carpal radiographs and lateral teleradiographs of males and females aged between 7 and 18 years. The carpal radiographs were used to determine the Carpal Maturation Index (CMI) and the lateral teleradiographs to determine the Vertebral Maturation Index (VMI). Each group of radiographs was examined and re-examined by 4 evaluators to analyze the reliability of each index, and a comparison was made between the BMI and VMI stages to assess the correlation between the indices. The results showed that there was no statistically significant difference between the 4 observers in the assessments of BMI and VMI, nor in the comparison between the indices mentioned. It can therefore be seen that 1) both the Carpal Maturation Index (CMI) and the Vertebral Maturation Index (VMI), according to the assessment methods proposed in this study, are reliable for assessing bone maturation in the population selected for the study, 2) there was a positive correlation between the two skeletal maturation indices assessed (CMI and VMI), 3) it is suggested that professionals should be cautious about considering the examination of the cervical vertebrae as an absolute method for assessing skeletal maturation in growing patients, as long as they are not familiar with the method.

Santos[35] in 2007 used 85 radiographs, 52 of which were of males and 33 of females, both with Down's syndrome. The aim was to check which of the methods: Greulich and Pyle, Eklof and Ringertz, Tanner and Whitehouse most closely matched chronological age in individuals with Down's syndrome, aged between 61 and 180 months, using hand and wrist radiographs. And observed that:

1) bone ages, according to the TW3 and Greulich and Pyle methods, are ahead of chronological age and there were no statistically significant differences between males and females;

2) bone ages, using the Eklof and Ringertz method, are delayed in relation to chronological age and there were statistically significant differences between female and male individuals; the TW3 and Greulich and Pyle bone age verification methods were statistically equal to each other and different from the Eklof and Ringertz method; and the TW3 and Greulich and Pyle methods are the closest to chronological ages, followed by Eklof and Ringertz.

Based on the results of the study by Moraes et al. 2008, skeletal age (SA) compared using the Greulich and Pyle method was delayed in relation to chronological age (CA) until the age of 7 for individuals with Down syndrome (DS), when compared to those without DS. However, the AS of individuals with DS advanced in relation to their chronological age (CA) at 15 years of age and therefore had a shorter period of skeletal development with early maturation compared to individuals without DS when skeletal maturation is usually around 18 years of age. The results of this study are important if patients with DS need orthodontic treatment, because the correct time for treating skeletal malocclusions depends on the individual's stage of skeletal maturation. In addition, the outcome of some treatment modalities, such as palatal expansion for correcting posterior crossbites, can be affected by an individual's stage of skeletal development.

2.3. Spinal development

In 1963 Bench[3] investigated the development of the cervical spine and its relationship with other bony structures in the face and with dental mineralization. He took measurements from the Frankfurt plane along a perpendicular that passed through the center of the cervical vertebrae. In the age range of seven to 12 years, 2.1, 2.2, 2.9 and 3.2 mm of growth in height per year from the second to the fifth cervical vertebrae respectively. He found that in the first two years of life, the morphology of the first, second and third cervical vertebrae is stable and concluded that the cervical vertebrae can be considered as a diagnostic parameter for orthodontic treatment.

In 1972 Lamparski[20] concluded that the cervical vertebrae routinely assessed using lateral teleradiographs were as clinically and statistically reliable in assessing skeletal age as the hand and wrist radiographic technique.

O'Reilly and Yanniello[29] in 1988 studied the relationship between bone maturation of the cervical vertebrae and changes in mandibular growth. They analyzed 13 lateral cephalometric radiographs of female subjects aged between 9 and 15 years. They used the average age at the stages of cervical bone development to create a curve that was superimposed on the pubertal growth curve. They observed that cervical vertebral maturation stages one, two and three appear before the peak of growth velocity, in the acceleration phase, while stages four and five appear after the peak, i.e. in the deceleration phase. They also pointed out that lateral cephalograms are as acceptable and valid as hand and wrist radiographs for analyzing bone age. They concluded that mandibular changes are statistically significant and correlate with the stages of bone development.

Hassel and Farman[17] in 1995 evaluated the skeletal maturation of the C2, C3 and C4 vertebrae, visualized in lateral cephalometric radiographs, and correlated it with the bone maturation of the hand and wrist. They pointed out that bone maturation is more closely related to sexual maturation than to height. They developed a vertebral maturation index divided into six distinct stages: initiation, acceleration, transition, deceleration, maturation and completion. They used 11 groups with ten females and ten males, totaling 220 patients. The age range used was between 8 and 18 years. They found that morphological changes in the vertebrae can denote the different stages of an individual's growth, making it a reliable method.

Garcia-Fernandez et al.[13] in 1998 determined the possible correlation between the bone maturation of the cervical vertebrae and the hand and wrist of 113 Mexican patients, fifty of whom were female and 63 male. The age range used was between 9 and 18 years, with all hand and wrist radiographs and lateral cephalometric radiographs taken on the same day. The methods used for analysis were Fishman (1982) for the phalanges and Hassel and Farman (1995) for the vertebrae. In all age groups, the correlation between the two methods was positive and high, with the age of 12 having the lowest percentage at 84.6%. They concluded that the hypothesis was true, since there was no difference between the methods applied to either females or males. They also stated that bone maturation of the cervical vertebrae is a neutral technique for different ethnic groups.

According to Román et al.[32] , in 2002, the method based on the morphological characteristics of the body of the cervical vertebrae can be used, instead of hand and wrist radiography, to designate the evolution of the individual's stage of maturation. In the sample investigated, Hassel and Farman's classification method[17] (1995) proved to be superior to Lamparski's method, since the latter was not sufficiently accurate to be used in male patients.

Also in 2002, Mito et al.[22] , established a new method for objectively assessing bone maturation using lateral cephalometric radiographs. They used the Tanner and Whitehouse method[38] (1983) in 66 female patients, while the analysis of bone ages by cervical vertebrae was evaluated in 176 females. The method used to obtain bone ages was by measuring the height and width of the vertebral bodies. They found that the correlation between bone age by hand and wrist and by maturation of the cervical vertebrae was statistically significant. They used the measurement of the vertebral bodies of C3 and C4 because they are easy to measure since C1 and C2 have a typical morphology which makes their analysis difficult. The difference between bone ages was small and statistically insignificant compared to chronological age. They concluded that in order to obtain bone age for the cervical vertebrae, it is feasible to carry out a detailed and objective study using cephalometric radiography.

Flores-Mir et al.[11] , 2006 evaluated 79 hand and wrist radiographs together with lateral cephalometric radiographs taken in male and female subjects and stated that the correlation between the stage of maturation through the evolution of the cervical vertebrae and hand and wrist indicated that the methods they used can be used in the different stages of skeletal maturation of individuals.

Morihisa[27] in 2005 evaluated the diagnosis, treatment plan and prognosis in the orthodontic treatment of children and adolescents, based on the degree of skeletal maturation and growth potential, with chronological and skeletal ages not always coinciding. To determine skeletal age, some methods can be used, such as carpal and cervical vertebrae radiography. The carpal radiograph is the oldest, providing a view of the hand and wrist region, where the indicators of maturity can be seen. The great concern related to simplifying diagnostic resources and reducing radiographic exposures of the patient has led researchers to analyze skeletal maturity using lateral cephalometric radiography, by visualizing the cervical vertebrae. In this study, the carpal and lateral cephalometric radiography methods are reviewed and compared in terms of their reliability and applicability for assessing skeletal maturation. The researched literature shows that both methods are in agreement when it comes to assessing skeletal maturation; however, the observation of the cervical vertebrae has been highly applicable, providing relevant diagnostic data for orthodontic practice.

Vieira et al.[41] in 2006 investigated the existence of differences in the effective length of the midface between male and female leucodermic individuals with Class I and Class II skeletal patterns, aged between seven and thirteen years and with the same stages of bone maturation of the cervical vertebrae. The sample consisted of 160 lateral cephalometric radiographs of individuals without previous orthodontic or facial orthopedic treatment. The results showed that there was no statistically significant difference between individuals with Class I skeletal pattern and Class II skeletal pattern, nor between males and females. Only the variation in CoA measurement in phase 1 (initiation) of cervical vertebral maturation was statistically lower than the other phases (2 = acceleration, 3 = transition and 4 = deceleration) in the two groups studied. We conclude that both male and female subjects with Class I and Class II skeletal patterns had similar effective midface lengths at the stages of bone maturation of the cervical vertebrae studied.

Caldas[4] in 2007 evaluated the applicability of the method for analyzing the bone age of the cervical vertebrae developed by Mito et al.[22] (2002) in Japanese girls in the Brazilian population, as well as establishing two new methods for Brazilian girls and boys, in order to objectively determine the skeletal maturation of the cervical vertebrae in lateral cephalometric radiographs. He used cephalometric radiographs and hand and wrist radiographs of 128 girls and 110 boys between the ages of 7 and 15.9 years, determined the bone age of the cervical vertebrae using the method of Mito et al.[22] , and the bone age was determined using the TW3 method. Bone age was used as the gold standard to determine the reliability of Mito's method. The third and fourth bodies of the cervical vertebrae were traced, measured and a regression formula was created in order to establish the bone age of the cervical vertebrae in Brazilian boys and girls. The results showed that there was a statistically significant difference between vertebral age and chronological age and between skeletal age and chronological age for the female population. In contrast, the male sample revealed a statistically significant difference between vertebral age and skeletal age and between vertebral age and chronological age. The creation of formulas for Brazilian boys and girls for the objective analysis of the skeletal maturation of the cervical vertebrae revealed no statistical difference between the bone age of the cervical vertebrae, skeletal age and chronological age, thus concluding that Mito's method can only be applied to Brazilian girls and that the formulas developed for the objective assessment of the bone age of the cervical vertebrae of Brazilian boys and girls are reliable and can be used.

In the study by Carinhena et al. 2014, the results revealed that adapting the methods developed by Martins and Sakima to assess skeletal maturation by cervical vertebrae in the pubertal growth spurt (PGS) curve is practical and useful in determining the stage of growth and development of individuals with Down syndrome. The stages of maturation assessed by the cervical vertebrae and ossification centers observed on the radiographs of the hand and wrist were considered reliable, with excellent agreement between the methods of Hassel and Farman as well as Baccetti, Franchi and McNamara Jr and Martins and Sakima. In addition, the results revealed an agreement ranging from reasonable to good for the three methods used to assess Down's skeletal maturation, showing statistical significance.

Chapter 3

3 PROPOSAL

The aim of this research is to

a)   to verify the applicability of the vertebral bone age assessment method developed by Caldas[4] for individuals without Down's syndrome, when applied to individuals with Down's syndrome.

b)   In the event of non-applicability, a formula will be created for obtaining bone age from the measurements of cervical vertebrae C3 and C4 on teleradiographs for people with Down's syndrome.

Chapter 4

4 MATERIAL AND METHOD

4.1 Sample

After being approved by the Research Ethics Committee under protocol number 018/2007-PH/CEP, one hundred and five medical records were selected from the archives of the Radiology Discipline of the Diagnosis and Surgery Department of the Institute of Science and Technology - ICT/Unesp, which were divided into 2 groups:

(Group I) Down's Syndrome: 57 records of individuals with Down's Syndrome, 23 female and 32 male.

(Group II) Control: 48 medical records of non-Down Syndrome individuals, 24 female and 24 male.

The two groups were made up of individuals aged between 5 and 18 years who had teleradiographs and hand and wrist radiographs taken on the same date.

4.2 Teleradiographs

Teleradiographs were used to analyze the vertebral bone age of the individuals, using the method proposed by Caldas[4] , which was created using Brazilian female and male individuals who did not have Down's syndrome.

This method consists of applying a formula for males and another for females, which uses mathematical ratios obtained by measuring variables in the bodies of the C3 and C4 cervical vertebrae to obtain the vertebral bone age of each individual.

Method proposed by Caldas[4] :

- Female vertebral bone age = 1.3523+6.7691x AH3/AP3 + 8.6408x AH4/AP4
- Male vertebral bone age = 1.4892+11.3736xAH3/AP3 + 4.8726x H4/AP4

For both cervical vertebrae, the following variables were obtained: (AH) anterior height of the vertebral body, (AP) anteroposterior width of the vertebral body and (H) height of the vertebral body, (PH) posterior height of the vertebral body. These variables were called AH3, AP3, H3, PH3 when referring to cervical vertebra C3; and AH4, AP4, H4, PH4 when referring to C4 (Figure 1).

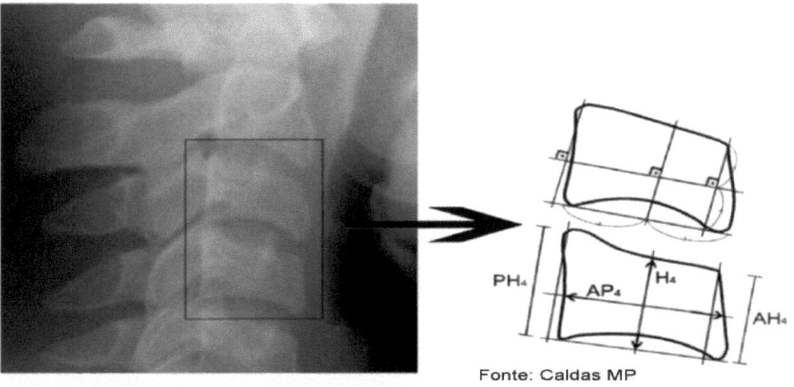

FIGURE 1: Body of the C3 and C4 cervical vertebrae measured using teleradiography: (AH) anterior height of the vertebral body, (AP) anteroposterior width of the vertebral body and (H) height of the vertebral body, (PH) posterior height of the vertebral body.

Source: Caldas MP

To obtain the variables, the bodies of the C3 and C4 cervical vertebrae were traced on acetate paper, and the variables were measured and applied to the formula.

To obtain the tracings, sheets of acetate paper (Microimage 4000) - Film Laser, 18 x 24 cm and 0.07 mm thick, were glued to the teleradiographs with the aid of 12 x 11 mm Scotch tape (3M) and placed on a negatoscope with two white fluorescent lamps of the same size at equal distances. To better visualize the teleradiographs, the tracings were taken in a dark room. To outline the anatomical structures, we used a pencil (Faber Castell poly super grip 0.5 mm) with graphite (Uni

2B 0.5 mm), a millimeter ruler (Desetec model 7130 - Trident) and an eraser (Carbex 40/20).

The segments of the C3 and C4 vertebrae were traced manually and measured using a millimeter ruler and a digital caliper. The C3 and C4 cervical vertebrae were traced on all the teleradiographs obtained from each individual. The tracings were repeated at least once a week, randomly, in order to obtain an average between the measurements obtained in each radiographic view and called vertebral bone age 1 and 2. This was done in order to minimize the possibility of error in the measurements. All measurements were made by a single, previously trained examiner, the author of this study.

4.3 Hand and wrist X-rays

The method proposed by Tanner and Whitehouse[39] (TW3) was used to obtain bone age from hand and wrist X-rays of the same individuals. This method visually assesses 13 ossification centers and their eight or nine stages of development, each with its own individual score. After the evaluation, the scores (Tables 1 and 2) are added up and the value compared with the respective bone age value in the table proposed by the author (Tables 3 and 4), considering males and females separately.

The 13 ossification centers proposed by the author are:
Radius, Ulna, Metacarpals I, III and V, Proximal Phalanges I, III and V, Middle Phalanges III and V and Distal Phalanges I, III and V (RUS method). For each of the thirteen ossification centers there are eight or nine stages of development (Figure 2).

Once the individual scores have been obtained (Tables 1 and 2), they are added together and the result is transformed into bone age using the proposed tables, considering gender separately (Tables 3 and 4).

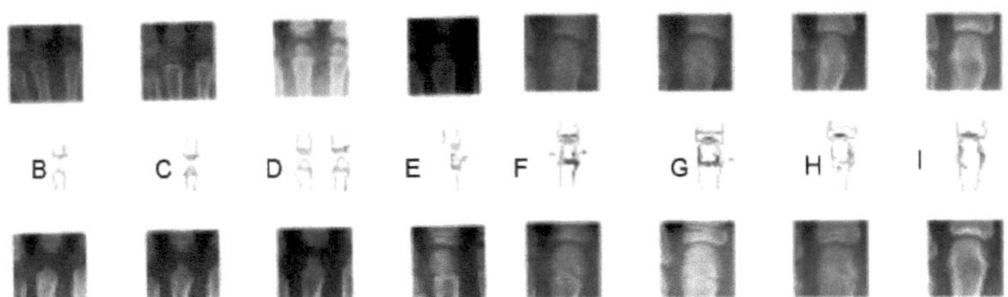

FIGURE 2 - Example of TW3 method scores - Stages of maturation

Table 1 - TW3 - RUS values for the scores obtained for **males .**

| | | | METACARPOS | | | FALANGES | | | | | | | |
| | | | | | | NEXT | | | AVERAGES | | DISTAILS | | |
Score	Radio	Ulna	MC I	MC III	MC V	Fp I	FP III	F P	Fm III	Fm V	Fd I	Fd III	Fd V
A	0	0	0	0	0	0	0	0	0	0	0	0	0
B	16	27	6	4	4	7	4	4	4	6	5	4	5
C	21	30	9	5	6	8	4	5	6	7	6	6	6
D	30	32	14	9	9	11	9	9	9	9	11	8	9
E	39	40	21	12	14	17	15	15	15	15	17	13	13
F	59	58	26	19	18	26	23	21	22	23	26	18	18
G	87	107	36	31	29	38	31	30	32	32	38	28	27
H	138	181	49	43	43	52	40	39	43	42	46	34	34
I	213	-	67	52	52	67	53	51	52	49	66	49	48

Table 2 - TW3 - RUS values for the scores obtained for females

			FALANGES

Score	Radio	Ulna	METACARPOS			NEXT			AVERAGES			DISTAILS	
			MC I	MC III	MC V	FP I	FP III	FP V	Fm III	Fm V	Fd I	Fd III	Fd V
A	0	0	0	0	0	0	0	0	0	0	0	0	0
B	23	30	8	5	6	9	5	6	6	7	7	7	7
C	30	33	12	8	9	11	7	7	8	8	9	8	8
D	44	37	18	12	12	14	12	12	12	12	15	11	11
E	56	45	24	16	17	20	19	18	18	18	22	15	15
F	78	74	31	23	23	31	27	26	27	28	33	22	22
G	114	118	43	37	35	44	37	35	36	35	48	33	32
H	160	173	53	47	48	56	44	42	45	43	51	37	36
I	218		67	53	52	67	54	51	52	49	68	49	47

Table 3 - Bone age estimated using the sum of the TW3 - RUS maturation score values for males

Score Maturapao	Bone Age (in years)	Score Maturapao	Bone Age (in years)	Score Maturapao	Bone Age (in years)
42	2.0	214	7.0	427	12.0
46	2.1	216	7.1	434	12.1
50	2.2	219	7.2	441	12.2
55	2.3	222	7.3	448	12.3
60	2.4	225	7.4	455	12.4

66	2.5	228	7.5	462	12.5
70	2.6	231	7.6	470	12.6
75	2.7	234	7.7	478	12.7
80	2.8	237	7.8	485	12.8
86	2.9	240	7.9	493	12.9
91	3.0	243	8.0	501	13.0
94	3.1	246	8.1	511	13.1
98	3.2	250	8.2	520	13.2
101	3.3	253	8.3	530	13.3
105	3.4	256	8.4	540	13.4
108	3.5	259	8.5	550	13.5
112	3.6	262	8.6	560	13.6
116	3.7	265	8.7	570	13.7
120	3.8	268	8.8	581	13.8
124	3.9	272	8.9	592	13.9
129	4.0	275	9.0	603	14.0
132	4.1	279	9.1	615	14.1
134	4.2	283	9.2	628	14.2
137	4.3	287	9.3	641	14.3
140	4.4	291	9.4	655	14.4
143	4.5	295	9.5	668	14.5
146	4.6	299	9.6	682	14.6
149	4.7	303	9.7	697	14.7
152	4.8	308	9.8	711	14.8
155	4.9	312	9.9	726	14.9
158	5.0	316	10.0	741	15.0
161	5.1	321	10.1	755	15.1
164	5.2	325	10.2	769	15.2
166	5.3	330	10.3	783	15.3
169	5.4	334	10.4	798	15.4
172	5.5	339	10.5	813	15.5
175	5.6	344	10.6	828	15.6
177	5.7	348	10.7	843	15.7
180	5.8	353	10.8	859	15.8
183	5.9	358	10.9	875	15.9
186	6.0	363	11.0	891	16.0
189	6.1	369	11.1	912	16.1
191	6.2	375	11.2	933	16.2
194	6.3	381	11.3	955	16.3
197	6.4	387	11.4	977	16.4
200	6.5	394	11.5	1000	16.5
202	6.6	400	11.6		
205	6.7	406	11.7		
208	6.8	413	11.8		
211	6.9	420	11.9		

Table 4 - Bone age estimated using the sum of the TW3 - RUS maturation score values for females

Score Maturapao	Bone age (in years)	Score Maturapao	Bone age (in years)	Score Maturapao	Bone age (in years)
126	2.0	335	7.1	695	12.2
130	2.1	339	7.2	705	12.3
134	2.2	343	7.3	714	12.4

139	2.3	347	7.4	724	12.5
143	2.4	351	7.5	735	12.6
148	2.5	355	7.6	745	12.7
153	2.6	359	7.7	755	12.8
158	2.7	363	7.8	766	12.9
163	2.8	367	7.9	776	13.0
168	2.9	372	8.0	787	13.1
174	3.0	377	8.1	798	13.2
178	3.1	382	8.2	809	13.3
182	3.2	387	8.3	820	13.4
186	3.3	393	8.4	832	13.5
191	3.4	398	8.5	843	13.6
195	3.5	404	8.6	855	13.7
200	3.6	409	8.7	867	13.8
204	3.7	415	8.8	879	13.9
209	3.8	421	8.9	891	14.0
214	3.9	427	9.0	902	14.1
219	4.0	434	9.1	912	14.2
222	4.1	441	9.2	923	14.3
225	4.2	448	9.3	933	14.4
228	4.3	455	9.4	944	14.5
231	4.4	462	9.5	955	14.6
234	4.5	470	9.6	966	14.7
238	4.6	478	9.7	978	14.8
241	4.7	485	9.8	989	14.9
244	4.8	493	9.9	1000	15.0
248	4.9	501	10.0		
251	5.0	509	10.1		
255	5.1	518	10.2		
258	5.2	526	10.3		
262	5.3	535	10.4		
265	5.4	543	10.5		
269	5.5	552	10.6		
273	5.6	561	10.7		
277	5.7	570	10.8		
281	5.8	579	10.9		
284	5.9	589	11.0		
288	6.0	597	11.1		
292	6.1	605	11.2		
296	6.2	614	11.3		
301	6.3	622	11.4		
305	6.4	631	11.5		
309	6.5	640	11.6		
313	6.6	649	11.7		
318	6.7	658	11.8		
322	6.8	667	11.9		
327	6.9	676	12.0		
331	7.0	685	12.1		

Example of the TW3 Method:

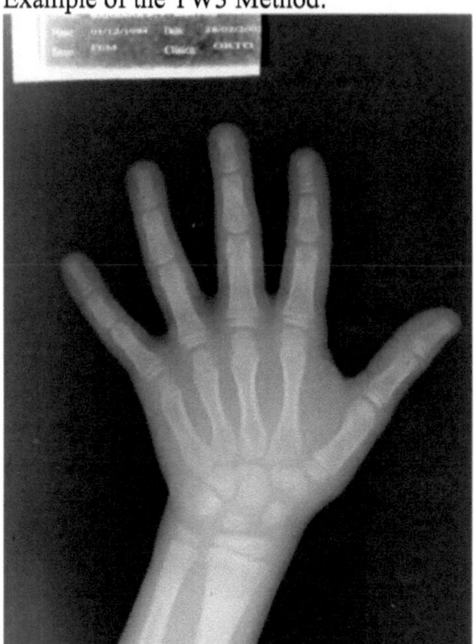

FIGURE 3- Radiograph of the hand and wrist of a male patient with Down's syndrome, with a chronological age of 9.42 years and a bone age of 7.5 years.

Table 5 - Analysis of the 13 ossification centers proposed by the method

| | | | METACARPOS | | | FALANGES | | | | | | | |
| | | | | | | NEXT | | | AVERAGES | | DISTAILS | | |
Esco re	Radio	Ulna	MC I	MC III	MC V	FP I	FP III	FP V	Fm III	Fm V	Fd I	Fd III	Fd V
A													
B													
C													
D	30	32											
E			21	12	14	17	15	15	15	15	17	13	13
F													

G													
H													
I													

By comparing the ossification centers obtained by radiographic analysis with the figures from the TW3 method (Figure 2), we have the scores for each corresponding ossification center. These scores are taken to Table 1 and compared to their respective numerical values. The sum of the numerical values is equal to 229. This, taken to Table 3, gives us a value for the individual's bone age of around 7 years and 5 months.

4.4 Statistical analysis of evaluations

The vertebral bone age obtained using the Caldas method[4] was compared with the bone age obtained using the Tanner and Whitehouse method[39] (TW3), and with the chronological age of the same individual, considering males and females separately, thus verifying the applicability of the Caldas method[4].

The FRIEDMAN and WILCOXON non-parametric tests were used for statistical analysis, and a significance level of 5% was set.

In view of the results obtained in this part of the research, we continue the proposition of this work by moving on to the item below.

4.5 Creation of a method for assessing vertebral bone age in individuals with Down's syndrome

Once the relative applicability of the Caldas method[4] for men only had been verified, it was possible to proceed with the second part of the proposal of this work. In this way, an objective method was created for women and another for men using Linear Regression.

Chapter 5

5 RESULTS AND DISCUSSION

This study used non-parametric statistical tests, which do not compare groups by mean but by data position. Even though the mean was not used for comparison, descriptive statistics were used to understand what happens in the results, as can be seen in Table 1, for non-Down syndrome patients.

Table 1 - Descriptive statistics for chronological, bone and vertebral bone ages for non-Down syndrome individuals.

Non-carriers of the syndrome	Male			Female		
	Chronological	Bone to	Vertebr al	Chronological	Bone	Vertebr al
Average	10,36	9,92	11,28	10,18	10,26	10,92
Median	10,42	10,30	11,02	10,42	10,00	10,55
Standard Deviation	2,83	2,12	1,88	1,75	1,23	1,89
CV	27,3%	21,3 %	16,6%	17,2%	12,0%	17,3%
Q1	9,17	8,25	10,22	9,00	9,55	9,79

Q3	11,75	11,30	12,32	11,17	10,70	11,61
N	25	25	25	25	25	25
IC	1,11	0,83	0,74	0,69	0,48	0,74
p-value	0,016			0,035		

In the group of non-Down syndrome patients, we found statistically significant differences between the ages of both males and females (Table 1). Therefore, in order to determine where this difference occurred, we used the Wilcoxon test to compare all the ages in pairs and thus find out exactly where the difference occurred.

Table 2 - p-values for non-Down syndrome patients.

Non-carriers of the syndrome		**Chronological**	**Bone**
Male	**Bone**	0,367	
	Vertebral	0,042	<0,001
Female	**Bone**	0,788	
	Vertebral	0,048	0,037

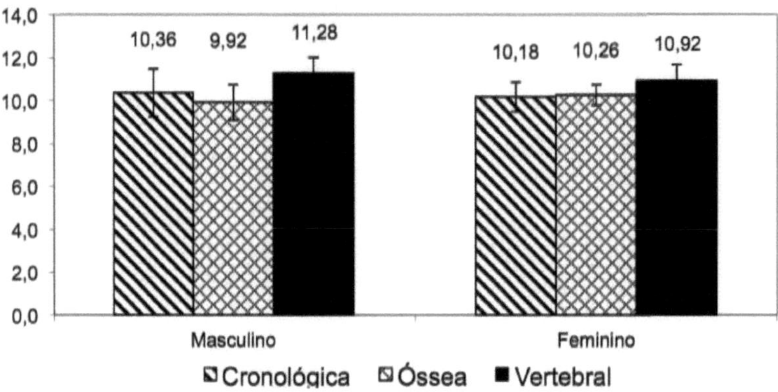

FIGURE 4- Comparison of chronological, bone and vertebral bone ages in non-Down syndrome patients.

Table 2 shows the p-values of the comparisons and shows that there is a statistically significant difference between vertebral bone age and chronological and bone age. For both males and females in the sample studied, vertebral bone age was higher than all other ages (Figure 4).

Next, we'll look at the results of the age comparison for the Down syndrome group.

Table 3 - Descriptive statistics for chronological, bone and vertebral bone ages for individuals with Down syndrome.

People with Down's syndrome	Male				Female			
	Chrono logic	Bone	Verte bral 1	Verte bral 2	Chrono logic	Bone	Verte bral 1	Verte bral 2
Average	13,05	13,00	13,30	13,52	11,68	11,37	12,38	12,86

Median	13,17	15,00	13,92	14,44	11,75	12,20	12,46	12,52
Deviation Standard	3,80	4,17	2,05	2,18	3,68	3,75	2,24	2,23
CV	29,1%	32,1%	15,4%	16,2%	31,5%	33,0%	18,1%	17,3%
Q1	10,79	10,00	11,50	11,80	9,00	8,98	10,27	11,17
Q3	16,08	16,50	14,79	14,99	14,04	15,00	13,59	14,32
N	35	35	35	35	23	23	23	23
IC	1,26	1,38	0,68	0,72	1,50	1,53	0,91	0,91
p-value	0,873				0,016			

Table 4 - p-values for people with Down's syndrome.

People with Down syndrome		Chronological	Bone	Vertebral 1
	Bone	0,308		
Female	**Vertebral 1**	0,287	0,114	
	Vertebral 2	**0,073**	**0,039**	**0,046**

Table 3 shows the group of Down's syndrome patients, for males and females. In the case of females, it was possible to see statistically significant differences between the ages, so when we looked at Table 4, we saw the p-values and identified that the difference occurred between vertebral bone age 2 and vertebral bone age 1. Vertebral bone age 2 is the one with the highest results compared to the other ages (Figure 5). Therefore, in this female sample of Down syndrome patients, the formula created by Caldas[4] was not applicable.

For male Down syndrome patients, there were no statistically significant differences between ages, as can be seen in Table 3 and Figure 5, so the formula created by Caldas[4] is applicable to this sample of individuals.

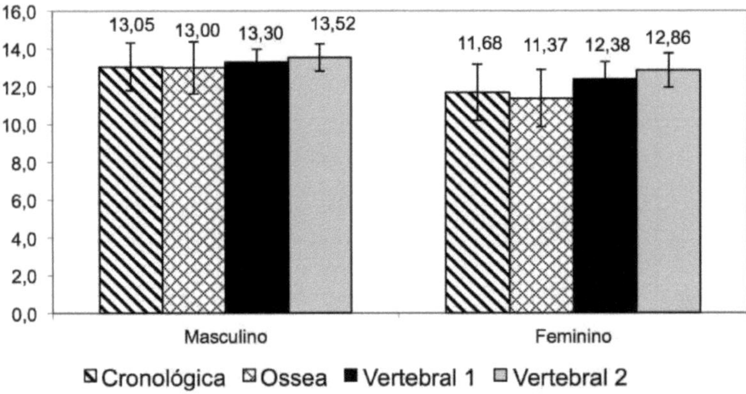

FIGURE 5- Comparison of chronological, bone, vertebral bone 1 and vertebral bone 2 ages in Down syndrome patients.

Based on these results, we move on to the next part of the proposal.

5.1 Presentation of the bone age method for people with Down syndrome.

With the data obtained, it was possible to prove that the formula created for Brazilian boys and girls by Caldas[4] was not applicable to female Down syndrome patients in the sample studied. Thus, two formula models were obtained, one for women and one for men. Table 5 shows the models generated and also the R^2 which assesses their quality.

Chart 5 - Final method for assessing bone age in Down syndrome patients.

We can see that both models are significant and well explanatory, i.e. they were well adjusted, as we can see from the R-value^2 . The Stepwise method was used in the development of the models. This method includes and excludes each variable until it is determined which are the most significant variables for explaining bone age. We applied the models found to the original data and obtained what we call the final bone age. We used the Wilcoxon test to compare the results between bone age (obtained by TW3) and vertebral bone age (obtained by Caldas[4]) with final bone age (calculated using the model developed in this study). This analysis was carried out only for people with Down's syndrome.

Chart 6 - Comparison of results between bone ages (TW3) and vertebral bone ages (Caldas[4]) and final bone ages in Down syndrome patients.

People with Down's syndrome	Male			Female		
	Final	Bone	Vertebral	Final	Bone	Vertebral
Average	13,00	13,00	13,30	11,36	11,37	12,38
Median	13,99	15,00	13,92	10,98	12,20	12,46
Standard Deviation	3,82	4,17	2,05	3,44	3,75	2,24
CV	29,4%	32,1%	15,4%	30,3%	33,0%	18,1%
Q1	10,20	10,00	11,50	9,18	8,98	10,27
Q3	16,00	16,50	14,79	14,18	15,00	13,59
N	35	35	35	23	23	23
IC	1,27	1,38	0,68	1,41	1,53	0,91

p-value	- x -	1	0,646	- x -	0,891	**0,024**

We found that the model is "applicable", as there are no statistically significant differences between the bone age value (obtained by TW3) and the final bone age calculated using the model.

It is worth noting that there is a difference between final bone age and vertebral bone age only among women.

The bone age index in Down's syndrome patients does not have a specific method for verification, which is of great importance, since according to García-Hoyos et al. (2017) Down's syndrome patients, in the presence of appropriate environmental factors, have a normal but small skeleton.

Applying three methods for estimating bone age in individuals with Down's syndrome, Santos[35] found statistical differences only in the Eklöf and Ringertz method, while with regard to gender and chronological age, the TW3 and Greulich and Pyle methods were statistically the same. In relation to the Eklöf and Ringertz method in patients with the syndrome, Sannomiya et al.[34] , observed the same, but found no statistically significant differences between the sexes.

Calles et al.[5] observed that the Greulich and Pyle method is used in people with Down's syndrome, but is not indicated for chronological ages: between 10 and 13 years for females and between 13 and 15 years for males, and concluded that between 10 and 13 years for females and between 13 and 15 years for males, there were statistically significant differences when analyzing chronological and bone age. The same conclusion was reached by Sannomiya et al.[33] , which is why we preferred to use the TW3 method in this study, as it is a more up-to-date method.

In this study, when we applied the TW3 method to people with Down's syndrome, we found no statistical differences between chronological and bone ages for males and females. However, Santos[35] , using the same TW3 method, found an average delay in chronological age in relation to bone age of 1.12 years for females and 1.31 years for males, i.e. bone ages were higher than chronological ages, but no statistically significant differences were found between males and females. However, he noted that the bone ages obtained using the TW3 and Greulich and Pyle methods were the closest to the chronological ages of these individuals.

Tavano[40] in 1976 found statistical differences between males and females. For individuals between the ages of 3 and 11, he observed advanced bone age, and between the ages of 12 and 17, delayed bone age, differences that can be explained by the fact that Tavano studied individuals who did not have Down's syndrome. Even though they studied individuals without Down's syndrome, Haiter Neto et al.[16] in 2000 found higher bone ages than chronological ages for both sexes, the same as Santos[35] 2007, in individuals with the syndrome. Guzzi et al.[14] in 2000, studying individuals who did not have the syndrome, also found that bone age was higher than chronological age for females, but that bone age was lower than chronological age for males.

Aguiar[2] , in 1998, analyzed the carpal and metacarpal bones of individuals with Down's syndrome and concluded that females had less bone development when compared to those without the syndrome and to syndromic males. Males with the syndrome had similar bone development to those without. We can therefore agree that there are differences in bone development, and according to the report by Carfi et al. 2017 there are also differences in bone mineral density.

The first person to demonstrate the applicability of the method of assessing the degree of skeletal maturation in teleradiographs was Lamparski[20] , who in 1972 observed changes in the size and shape of the cervical vertebrae and compared them with radiographs of the hand and wrist, assessed by Greulich and Pyle[15] in 1959. Based on the morphological changes in the cervical vertebrae C2 to C6, he described six stages of maturation.

Hassel and Farman[17] , 1995 found a high correlation between the indicators studied by Lamparski[20] , and modified the original method, proposing the evaluation of images corresponding to the C2, C3 and C4 vertebrae, due to the fact that they were not covered by the thyroid protector during the radiographic incidence.

Román et al.[32] , in the population investigated (Spanish children) observed that the Hassel and Farman classification[17] can be used to estimate the stage of maturation in males and females, while the Lamparski classification[20] is unreliable in this population for males.

Morishia[27] in 2005, concluded that the carpal method and the cervical vertebrae are in agreement when it comes to verifying skeletal maturation, and the use of teleradiography is important due to the reduced exposure of patients to X-rays, as well as the lower cost.

Damian et al.[7] in 2006, agree with this regarding the verification of skeletal maturation, but suggest caution when examining the cervical vertebrae if the examiner is not familiar with them.

Mito et al.[22] used teleradiographs of Japanese women to create a formula using the measurements of the C3 and C4 vertebral bodies to obtain the bone age of the cervical vertebrae in these individuals. They concluded that this result is reliable when compared to the one obtained by hand and wrist radiography using the TW2 method. In 2007, Caldas[4] applied the formula of Mito et al.[22] to Brazilian males and females, and observed that it was only applicable to Brazilian girls. He then created a formula for analyzing the skeletal maturation of the cervical vertebrae in Brazilian boys and girls.

As no studies were found in the literature on the maturation of the cervical vertebrae in individuals with Down's syndrome, the comparison was made with patients without the syndrome. And according to the study by Moraes et al. 2008, there is a difference where those with Down syndrome (DS) had a shorter period of skeletal development with early maturation when compared to individuals without DS.

Also in the study by Carfi et al. 2017, we can observe a difference in bone mineral density between Down syndrome carriers and non-carriers, and Looker et al. 2012, Woodson 2000 and Fink et al. 2008, observed that variation in bone mineral density occurs between genders in Down individuals.

In this study, we applied the Caldas formula,[4] created for male and female Brazilians, to non-Down syndrome patients, and the results differed from those of the author, as the formula created was not statistically significant in our sample. And when applied to the sample of people with Down's syndrome, it was only statistically significant for males and not for females.

In view of these results, an objective method was created using measurements of the C3 and C4 cervical vertebrae obtained from teleradiography to obtain the bone age of patients with Down's syndrome. We believe that this method can contribute to the analysis of bone age in these patients.

CONCLUSION

According to the methodology used, we can conclude that:

a) the method proposed by Caldas[4] when applied to our sample of female and male individuals not suffering from Down's syndrome, showed statistically significant differences between bone, chronological and vertebral bone ages. We noticed that for both females and males, vertebral bone age was older than the other ages.

b) when applied to female subjects with Down syndrome, the statistically significant difference is between vertebral bone age and bone age. Vertebral bone age is also older than other ages.

c) the same method showed no statistically significant differences between bone age, vertebral bone age and chronological age in males with Down syndrome.

d) due to the fact that the method analyzed is not applicable to females, we created an objective method to obtain the value of vertebral bone age in male and female Down syndrome patients, through measurements of the C3 and C4 cervical vertebrae using teleradiography.

REFERENCES

Acheson RM, Vinicius JH, Fower GB. Studies in the reliability of assessing skeletal maturity from x- rays. 3. Greulich-Pyle and TannerWhitehouse method contrasted. Hum Biol. 1966 Sept; 38(3):204-18.

Aguiar SMHCA. Bone development of children with Down syndrome: radiographic morphometric study of carpal and metacarpal bones [thesis]. Arapatuba: Arapatuba Dental School, São Paulo State University;1998.

Bench RW. Growth of the cervical vertebrae as related to tongue, face, and denture behavior. Am J Orthod.1963 Mar; 49(3):183-214.

Caldas MP. Evaluation of skeletal maturation in the Brazilian population by analyzing the cervical vertebrae [thesis]. Piracicaba: Piracicaba School of Dentistry, State University of Campinas; 2007.

Calles AC, Carinhena G. Assessment of bone age in individuals with Down's syndrome using radiographs of the hand and wrist.

Carinhena G, Siqueira DF, Sannomiya EK. Skeletal maturation in individuals with Down's syndrome: comparison between PGS curve, cervical vertebrae and bones of the hand and wrist. Dental Press J Orthod. 2014 Jul-Aug;19(4):58-65.

Carfi A, Liperoti R, Fusco D, Giovannini V, Brandi V, Vetrano DL, Meloni E, Mascia D, Villani ER, Manes Gravina E, Bernabei R, Onder G. Bone mineral density in adults with Down syndrome. Osteoporos Int (2017) 28:2929-2934. doi:10.1007/s00198-017-4133-x.

7th Symposium on Informatics in Orthodontics and Functional Jaw Orthopedics; Oct 9-12, 2004; Sao Paulo. [access in: mar.2008]. Available at: http: // www.cleber.com.br/orto2004/andreia.html

Coelho CRS, Loevy HT. Dental aspects of Down's syndrome. Ars Curandi Odontol. 1982; 8(3): 9-16.

Damian MF, Woitchunas FE, Cericato GO, Cechinato F, Moro G, Massochin ME, Castoldi FL . Reliability and correlation analysis of two skeletal maturation estimation indices: carpal index and vertebral index. Rev Dental Press Ortodon Ortop Facial. 2006 Sep/Oct;11(5):110-20.

Eklöf O, Ringertz H. A method for assessment of skeletal maturity. Ann Radiol. 1967;10(3):330-36.

Ferreira NSP, Aguiar SA, Santos - Pinto R. Prevalence of permanent tooth agenesis in Down syndrome patients. Radiographic study. Rev Inst Cienc Saúde.1993 Jul/ Dec;11(2):57-61.

Ferreira NSP, Aguiar SA, Santos - Pinto R. Frequency of dental gyroversion in patients with Down syndrome. Clinical study. Rev Robrac. 1998; 7 (23):24-6.

Fink HA, Harrison SL, Taylor BC, Cummings SR, Schousboe JT, Kuskowski MA, Stone KL, Ensrud KE (2008) Study of Osteoporotic Fractures (SOF) Group. Differences in site-specific fracture risk among older women with discordant results for osteoporosis at hip and spine: study of osteoporotic fractures. J Clin Densitom 11:250-259

Flores-mir C, Burgess CA, Champney M, Jensen RJ, Pitcher MR, Major PW. Correlation of skeletal maturation stages determined by cervical. Vertebrae and hand-wrist evaluations. Angle Orthod. 2006;76(1):1-5.

Freitas JAS, Lopes ES, Tavano O. Correlation between methods of determining biological age. J. Pediatr. 1990;66:56-60.

Garcia-Fernandez P, Torre H, Flores L, Rea J. The cervical vertebrae as maturational indicators. J Clin Orthod.1998 Apr;32(4):221-25.

García-Hoyos M García-Unzueta MT,Luis D, Valero C, Riancho JA. Diverging results of areal and volumetric bone mineral density in Do wn syndrome. Osteoporos Int. 2017 Mar;28(3):965-972. doi: 10.1007/S00198-016-3814-1.

Guzzi BSS, Carvalho LS. Study of bone maturation in young patients of both sexes using hand and wrist radiographs. Rev Dental Press Ortodon Ortop Maxilar. 2000 Sep./Dec;33(3):49-58.

Greulich WW, Pyle SI. Radiographic atlas of skeletal development of the hand and wrist. Stanford: Stanford University Press; 1959.

Haiter-Neto F, Almeida SM, Leite CC. Comparative study of the Greulich & Pyle and Tanner & Whitehouse bone age estimation methods. Pesqui Odontol Bras. 2000;14(4):378-84.

Hala LA, Moraes MEL, Villapa-Carvalho MFL, de Castro Lopes SLP, Gamba TO. Comparison of accuracy between dental and skeletal age in the estimation of chronological age of Down syndrome individuals. Forensic Sci Int. 2016 Sep;266:578.e1-578.e10. doi: 10.1016/j.forsciint.2016.06.019.

Hassel B, Farman AG. Skeletal maturation evolution using cervical vertebral. Am J Orthod Dentofac Orthop. 1995;107(1):58-66.

Kimura K. Growth of the second metacarpal according to chronological age and skeletal maturation. Anat Rec. 1976 Feb;184(2):147-57.

Kurita LM. Applicability of methods for estimating bone and dental age in Brazilians from Ceará [thesis]. Piracicaba: Piracicaba School of Dentistry, State University of Campinas; 2004.

Lamparski D. Skeletal age assessment utilizing cervical vertebrae [thesis]. Pittsburg (USA): University of Pittsburg; 1972.

Looker AC, Melton LJ, Borrud LG, Shepherd JA. Lumbar spine bone mineral density in US adults: demographic patterns and relationship with femur neck skeletal status. Osteoporos Int (2012) 23:1351-1360. doi :10.1007/s00198-011-1693-z .

Marshall D. Radiographic correlation of hand, wrist, and tooth development. Dent Radiogr Photogr. 1976;49(3):51-72.

Mito T, Sato K, Mitani H. Cervical vertebral bone age in girls. Am J Orthod Dentofac Orthop. 2002;122(4):380-85.

Moraes LC, Médici Filho E, Castilho JCM, Leonelli, ME. Bone age. RGO. 1994 Jul/Aug;42(4):201-03.

Moraes MEL, Tanaka JL, Moraes LC, Filho EM, Melo Castilho JC. Skeletal age of individuals with Down syndrome. Spec Care Dentist. 2008 May-Jun;28(3):101-6. doi: 10.1111/j.1754-4505.2008.00020.x.

Moraes MEL. Verification of bilateral developmental asymmetry using hand and wrist radiographs, based on bone age assessment [dissertation]. Sâo José dos Campos: Sâo José dos Campos School of Dentistry, São Paulo State University; 1995.

Moraes MEL. Pubertal growth spurt - relationship between dental mineralization, chronological age, dental age and bone age: radiographic method [thesis]. São José dos Campos: Sâo José dos Campos School of Dentistry, São Paulo State University; 1997.

Moraes LC, Médici-Filho E, Moraes MEL, Castilho JCM, Dotto PP, Dotto GN. Occurrence of taurodontism in individuals with Down syndrome. Rev Inst Cienc Saúde. 2004;22(4):317-22.

Morihisa O, Feres R, Vasconcelos MHF, Sannomiya EK. Skeletal maturation assessment: a comparative review of the carpal method and cervical vertebrae imaging. Orthodontics SPO. 2005 Jul/Sep;38(3):70- 7.

Moyers RE. Basic concepts of growth and development. Rio de Janeiro: Guanabara Koogan; 1991.

O'Reilly MT, Yanniello GJ. Mandibular growth changes and maturation of cervical vertebrae: a longitudinal cephalometric study. Angle Orthod.1988 Apr;58(2):179-84.

Papich D, Lazzari CM, Golendziner S, Chiappetta ALML. Study of chewing and dental occlusion in individuals with Down syndrome. Rev Int Odonto-Psicol Odontol Pacientes Especiais. 2005;1(1):86-90.

Rey SC, Fazzi R, Birman EG. Main craniofacial alterations in Down syndrome patients. Rev. Fac. Odontol. 1991;3(1):59-64.

Roman PS, Palma JC, Oteo MD, Nevado E. Skeletal maturation determined by cervical vertebrae development. Eur Orthod. 2002;24:303-11.

Sannomiya EK, Médici-Filho E, Castilho JCM, Graziosi MAOC. Assessment of bone age in individuals with Down syndrome using hand and wrist radiographs. Rev. Odontol. Unesp. 1998;27(2):527-36.

Sannomiya EK, Calles A. Comparison of bone age with chronological age in individuals with Down syndrome by the Eklof & Ringertz index, using hand and wrist radiographs. Cienc Odontol Bras. 2005;8(2):39-44.

Santos LRA. Comparative analysis of three methods for estimating bone age in individuals with Down syndrome, using hand and wrist radiographs [thesis]. Sao José dos Campos: Sao José dos Campos School of Dentistry, São Paulo State University; 2007.

Silva KG, Aguiar SMHCA. Dental eruption in children with Down syndrome and phenotypically normal children: a comparative study. Revista Odontol Araçatuba. 2003 Jan/Jul;24(1):33-9.

Tanner JM, Whitehouse RH. Standards for skeletal age. Institute of Child Health. London: University of London; 1959.

Tanner JM, Whitehouse RH, Cameron N. Assessment of skeletal maturity and prediction of adult height (TW2 Method). Institute of Education, University of London: Academic Press; 1983.

Tanner JM, Whitehouse RH, Cameron N, Healy MJR, Goldstein H.

Assessment of skeletal maturity and prediction of adult height (TW3 Method). Australas Radiol. 2003,47:340-41.

Tavano O. Estudo das principais tabelas de avaliação da idade biológica, através do desenvolvimento osseo, visando sua aplicação em brasileiros leucodermas da regiao de Bauru [thesis]. Bauru: Bauru School of Dentistry; University of Sao Paulo; 1976.

Vieira AM, Carlos RG, Paula AV, Bothrel JRS, Armond MC, Ribeiro A. Lateral cephalometric evaluation of skeletal Class I and II individuals with bone maturation of the cervical vertebrae. Rev. Dent Press Ortodon Ortop Facial. 2006 Nov/Dec;11(6):62-72.

Woodson G (2000) Dual X-ray absorptiometry T-score concor- dance and discordance between the hip and spine measurement sites. J Clin Densitom 3:319-324.

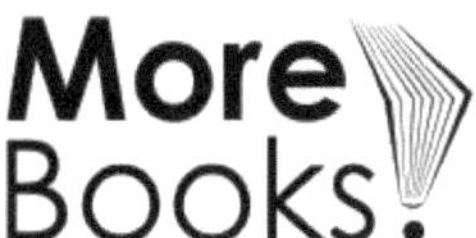

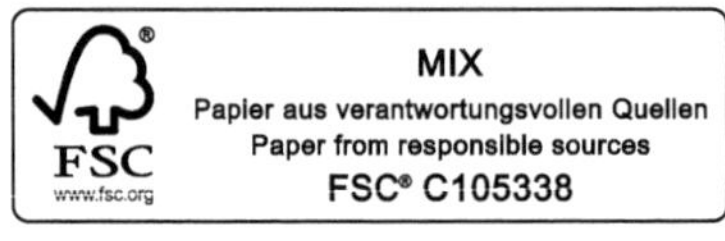

Printed by Books on Demand GmbH, Norderstedt / Germany